VAGUS NERVE

Discover Your Body's Natural Healing Body Switch

Includes Exercises To Activate Your Vagus Nerve, Reduce Inflammation, Anger, Chronic Illness, PTDS And Vertigo.

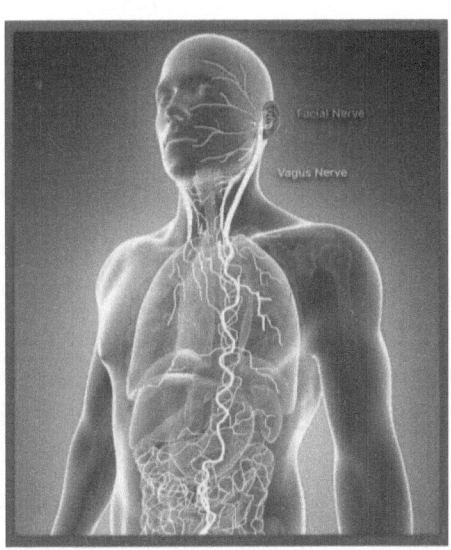

Michael D. Kaiser

VAGUS NERVE

Discover Your Body's Natural Healing Body Switch

Copyright © 2020, 2024 - Michael D. Kaiser.
All rights reserved.

No part of this guide may be reproduced in any form without permission in writing from the publisher except in the case of brief quotations embodied in critical articles or reviews.

Published by:

Dana Publishing
12804 Chillicothe Road #202
Chesterland, Ohio 44026
USA

The information contained in this book and its contents is not designed to replace or take the place of any form of medical or professional advice; and is not meant to replace the need for independent medical, financial, legal or other professional advice or services, as may be required. The content and information in this book has been provided for educational and entertainment purposes only.

The content and information contained in this book has been compiled from sources deemed reliable, and it is accurate to the best of the Author's knowledge, information and belief. However, the Author cannot guarantee its accuracy and validity and cannot be held liable for any errors and/or omissions. Further, changes are periodically made to this book as and when needed. Where appropriate and/or necessary, you must consult a professional (including but not limited to your doctor, attorney, financial advisor or such other professional advisor) before using any of the suggested remedies, techniques, or information in this book.

You agree that by continuing to read this book, where appropriate and/or necessary, you shall consult a professional (including but not limited to your doctor, attorney, or financial advisor or such other advisor as needed) before using any of the suggested remedies, techniques, or information in this book.

This book is not giving official medical advice; please consult your primary care doctor for medical related questions.

Table of Contents

Introduction……………………………………………………..6

    The Vagus Nerve And Hunger…………………………………8

Chapter 1: Vagus nerve explained…………………………184

    Functions of vagus nerve…………………………………206

    Branches of vagus nerve…………………………………228

    Most important branches……………………………………239

Symptoms of vagus nerve compression……………………..23

    Vagus disease…………………………………………31

    How to know that the vagus nerve needs to be tuned…………32

    How the magical vagus nerve helps our body to calm down…..33

Lack of social interaction……………………………………30

Chapter 2: The science………………………………………..32

    The role of the vagus nerve………………………………….33

    Origin of vagus nerve…………………………………..35

    Where the vagus nerve is located………………………….36

    Vagus nerve path…………………………………………37

    Vasovagal SYNCOPE………………………………………39

Chapter 3: What happens when it malfunctions………………51

    How To Diagnose Vagus Nerve Damage……………………51

    Symptoms Of Vagus Nerve Dysfunction……………………55

Chapter 4: Common problems it can heal……………………..60

Dangers..63

Medical procedure dangers...66

How to plan...66

Nourishment and drugs...66

What you can anticipate..66

During the technique...66

Vagus Nerve Stimulation (VNS) Dramatically Reduces Arthritic Inflammation..72

How improving your vagal tone can prevent physical inflammation...75

Chapter 5: PTSD...79

Chapter 6: Causes of anxiety, depression and inflammation.....88

What are the most well-known anxiety disorders?..................92

Chapter 7: How to activate your vagus nerve.....................103

Conclusion..111

Appendix..113

Introduction

Your body's Guardian Angel?

Within the deep network of your nervous system lies a remarkable structure, the Vagus nerve. Stretching from the brainstem down to the abdomen, this nerve is not just a mere bundle of fibers; it's a multifaceted regulator that influences a plethora of bodily functions, from digestion to emotional well-being.

Did you know it has a profound impact on human health?

Have you at any point asked why some people feel full after eating very little or a small meal, and other individuals are super hungry after eating a major serving?

The reason may be in the condition and health of your vagus nerve. The vagus nerve is directly responsible for your digestion system, stomach function (slow or fast emptying) and appetite.

The vagus nerve, scientifically known as the cranial nerve X, is one of the longest and most complex nerves in the body. It serves as a vital link between the brain and various organs, including the heart, lungs, stomach, and intestines.

This cranial nerve acts as a bi-directional communication channel, continuously relaying information back and forth between the brain and the body's internal organs.

One of the vagus nerve's primary roles is in the parasympathetic nervous system, which governs the body's rest-and-digest response.

When activated, the vagus nerve initiates a cascade of physiological responses that promote relaxation and restoration. It slows down the heart rate, enhances digestion, and stimulates the release of enzymes and acids in the stomach to facilitate nutrient absorption; essentially putting the body in a state of optimal functioning.

But the vagus nerve's influence extends far beyond basic bodily functions. Recent research has uncovered its profound impact on mental health and emotional well-being. This nerve serves as a crucial component of the brain-gut axis, a bidirectional communication system between the gastrointestinal tract and the brain. Through this pathway, the vagus nerve plays a crucial role in regulating mood, stress responses, and even social behavior.

Furthermore, the vagus nerve is intricately involved in the body's inflammatory response. By modulating the release of cytokines and other inflammatory mediators, it helps to regulate the immune system's response to infection and injury.

Dysfunction of the vagus nerve has been linked to various inflammatory disorders, including rheumatoid arthritis, inflammatory bowel disease, and depression.

Interestingly, the vagus nerve's influence extends beyond the confines of the body, affecting our social interactions and interpersonal relationships.

Known as the "social nerve," it plays a crucial role in regulating our ability to empathize, connect with others, and form meaningful bonds. Studies have shown that individuals with stronger vagal tone – a measure of the vagus nerve's activity – tend to have better social skills and interpersonal relationships.

Moreover, the vagus nerve has garnered attention in the field of bioelectronics medicine, where researchers are exploring its potential for treating a wide range of disorders.

By stimulating or modulating the activity of the vagus nerve through electrical impulses, scientists have achieved remarkable results in treating conditions such as epilepsy, depression, and even obesity.

The vagus nerve shows how interconnected the human body and mind are. From regulating basic bodily functions to influencing our emotional well-being and social interactions, this master nerve plays a pivotal role in shaping our health and overall quality of life. As our understanding of its capabilities continues to evolve, the vagus nerve holds the promise of unlocking new avenues for treating and managing a myriad of health conditions, paving the way for a healthier and more harmonious future

The vagus nerve is a trunk-line nerve that associates your gut to your brain, and it's a significant part of the parasympathetic sensory system (the "rest and summary" reaction, essentially something contrary to "fight or flight").

All signals going up from the gut to the brain through the vagus nerve influences your feeling of satiation or having more cravings, as well as your mood and feelings of anxiety, and the initiation of your inflammatory stress reaction.

Signals running down the vagus nerve from the brain to the gut influence digestion, discharge of stomach related compounds, and gastrointestinal motility (that is an extravagant word for where you are on the scale from constipation to looseness of the bowels).

It's an extremely significant pathway, and vagus nerve initiation is also associated with obesity, gastrointestinal illnesses, cardiovascular illnesses, disposition issues like depression, and a wide range of other incessant medical issues. Here's a look at why the vagus nerve is so significant, and how your eating routine can improve your wellbeing by influencing vagal nerve signals from the gut.

The Vagus Nerve And Hunger

One significant kind of correspondence with the vagus nerve is craving and hunger signals.

For instance...

The stomach sends the fullness satiety flag up the vagus nerve to your brain. This is the how your brain knows to quit feeling hungry after a meal.

The synapses detect nutrients delivered in the gut, similar to serotonin and ghrelin, can likewise send the yearning and satiety flag up the vagus nerve to the brain.

Obesity is related with a lower sensitivity of the vagus nerve to completion signals, and there's a great deal of proof this is caused explicitly by your eating routine.

Obesity inciting diets can really adjust the affectability of the vagus nerve to completion signals, so it takes more nourishment for your brain to get the "full currently" signal. Also, much the same as you may expect, invigorating the vagus nerve (to "increase the volume" on the satiety signal) will in general cause weight reduction in test animals – despite the fact that it's significant that tests in people have mixed outcomes.

The Vagus Nerve and Other Health Issues

Appetite is one integral motivation behind why the vagus nerve is significant. However, in the event that you bring a jump into PubMed, you'll see that vagus nerve damage is really connected with a wide range of different issues. That is on the grounds that the vagus nerve likewise manages irritation, and aggravation is engaged with pretty much every chronic ailment. Invigorating vagus nerve signals to the brain are calming – it flags the brain to turn down the stress reaction and lessens the generation of inflammatory cytokines.

The impacts here are somewhat difficult to unravel in light of the fact that the vagus nerve is a two-way street and there are a ton of convoluted input circles between the brain and the gut (recall that the vagus nerve runs in two different directions!). Be that as it may, for individuals who simply care about improving their wellbeing, the correct system may be less significant than the outcomes, which are certainly noteworthy:

- Vagus nerve control of inflammation influences cardiovascular wellbeing, and vagus nerve stimulation may help counteract cardiovascular events.

- Vagus nerve flagging is lost in patients with Crohn's Disease (a type of Inflammatory Bowel Disease), and one little, starter focus found that vagal nerve stimulation helps treat the indications.

- The vagus nerve may likewise be involved with Irritable Bowel Syndrome, and vagal stimulation may be useful for diminishing IBS pain.

- This study is truly intriguing: treating diabetes-inclined rodents with vagal nerve stimulation forestalls both anxiety and insulin resistance. That is a gigantic bit of proof that depression and diabetes may both have their start in the gut.

And when a terrible eating routine is influencing the affectability of your vagus nerve, it could likewise affect every one of these ailments. This could be one motivation behind why gut wellbeing is such a major player in generally addressing wellbeing.

Care and Feeding of your Vagus Nerve

Up until now, we realize that an obesogenic "cafeteria diet" (high-fat, high-carb shoddy nourishment) diminishes the affectability of the vagus nerve, and that vagus nerve stimulation neutralizes that, with enormous advantages for weight... and for pretty much everything else. Unfortunately, the "vagal nerve stimulation" in these specific studies isn't something you can do at home; they used a gadget that was carefully embedded in the subjects' bodies.

However, when a lousy eating routine can lessen the sensitivity and affectability of the vagus nerve, possibly a decent healthy diet can help reestablish it. Other than "don't eat a low quality nourishment diet," there's somewhat progressively more explicit research than this.

This study found that dietary fat decreased stress through its impacts on the vagus nerve. The creators inferred that "high-fat... sustenance is possibly remedial in other heated issues, for example, sepsis and inflammatory bowel disease (IBD) portrayed by an inflammatory reaction in which... intestinal obstruction capacity is disabled."

That is upheld up by the association between a ketogenic (exceptionally high-fat, low-carb) diet and vagal nerve stimulation as two viable treatments for treatment-safe epilepsy. It's conceivable that a ketogenic diet have a portion of its craving stifling, calming impacts through invigorating the vagus nerve.

This study additionally found that a probiotic (Lactobacillus casei strain Shirota) actuated the vagus nerve. The probiotic changed the gut-to-brain stress motioning in understudies taking a painful test and suppressed the arrival of the stress hormone cortisol. That proposes that probiotics may have the option to break the gut-brain input cycle in the places the vagus nerve where mental pressure messes the gut up, which sends increasing hormonal pressure signals to the brain, which cause more gut issues.

High-impact exercise may be useful.

For instant results, you can likewise do your very own vagal nerve stimulation utilizing the Valsalva move. Drop down, take a full breath, and afterward close your mouth and squeeze your nose shut with the goal that no air can get away. At that point imagine you're attempting to inhale out, yet without opening your nose or mouth – you should feel the weight from the air. Continue doing this for 15-20 seconds, and afterward let the let some circulation in and inhale normally. (And when you do any weightlifting, this is the kind of breath-holding you do to settle your spine during overwhelming squats and deadlifts.)

The Valsalva move doesn't have long-term impacts, however it may be useful for a quick circumstance, similar to directly before a test or during an unpleasant drive.

That is not a great deal to go on – there simply aren't many studies on eating regimen and the vagus nerve. In any case, it's something to start with, and it backs up the significant ways that the gut, the brain, and the remainder of your body are altogether linked. Thinking about the vagus nerve clarifies why gut wellbeing, psychological wellness, and entire body wellbeing are so tangled up with one another, and why great gut wellbeing is so significant for things process well in the body as a whole.

Chapter 1: The Vagus Nerve Explained

The vagus nerve manages so many parts of the body that it can be devastating when something goes wrong with it. If there is anything that damages the nerve, such as medication, trauma, or disease; can the body heal itself or are you stuck with nerve damage for the rest of your life?

It really all depends on how bad the damage is. Nerve damage is notorious for being slow to heal and the vagus nerve is no exception. However, scientists have tested the ability of the vagus nerve to regenerate in rats and the results have been surprising. Not only have vagus nerve techniques helped with the restoration of the central vagal parts, but they have also been shown to increase synaptic plasticity. This means that even when the brain suffers damage from damage done to the vagus nerve, it can be reversed, to a certain extent.

In tests done on rats, it took roughly 4.5 months to regenerate the central vagal nerve. That's good news for people, though it hasn't been fully tested in humans. However, studies have also shown that rebuilding the nerves in the gastrointestinal tract did not occur over the course of 45 weeks, or almost a year, which is how long the study lasted. It will definitely take time for nerves to grow back and regenerate, but the fact that it is actually possible is very promising.

While the central sections of the vagal nerve can be regenerated surprisingly quickly, it takes much longer to regrow the areas that branch out from it. It's important to note this because you shouldn't expect instant results from the exercises and techniques given in this book. It takes time to heal nerve damage, and that means you need to be patient and consistent if you have suffered from vagal nerve damage. Stimulation of the vagus nerve can help it grow and recover from damage. Again, it takes time, but if you are willing to put in the time and effort, you'll find that things gradually get better. As many people have discovered before you, this is not a trick. Vagus nerve stimulation really works and it can have an incredible impact on your life.

Many people that suffered various ailments were able to reverse them through vagus nerve stimulation, and it really does seem like a miracle, but it's actually just the science of the nervous system doing its job.

With the right stimulation, your vagus nerve will start working better than ever and becomes even more efficient too. Even if you haven't suffered from any particular trauma or nerve damage, you can still expect some results from toning up your vagus nerve. It can only help you feel better and ensure that your body runs more efficiently. The amount of energy you'll have will increase and you will find that it is easier to live the lifestyle you want. There's an amazing amount of information out there if you know what to look for, yet it's still not common knowledge. This alone is amazing, but here you'll learn the basics to get started now and how to stimulate your vagus nerve to start the process of recovery.

Functions of vagus nerve

Vagus nerve: In addition to the muscle movement and sensation of the pharyngeal head and throat, it has a regulating effect on the autonomic nerves distributed in the internal organs such as the heart, respiratory organs, and digestive organs, as well as the function of the secretory gland and the expansion and contraction of smooth muscle.

The amount of breathing is large and slow, and the activity of the parasympathetic nervous system can be enhanced by activating the vagus nerve. It can strengthen the sympathetic nervous system and thus the brainwaves of the brain.

It can activate the hypothalamus in the brain and regulate various regions of the cerebral cortex. It can trigger a positive physiological process because it activates the vagus nerve that controls our internal organs.

The activation of the vagus nerve moves upward through the nucleus of the brain stem into the brain, and the message is transmitted along two paths. One of the pathways leads up to the brain regions of the cerebral cortex via the hypothalamus

The frontal cortex can calm the over-activated brain area and reduce anxiety; the passage to the parietal lobe and occipital lobe can coordinate the rhythm of the sensory and motor cortex, increase attention and alertness, and calm the mind.

The other path affects the brain regions associated with our emotions via the neural pathways that enter and exit the limbic system of the brain. The main role of the vagus nerve is to control our heart, lungs, digestive organs and glands. However, it is currently considered to be only 20% of the vagus nerve function.

In fact, 80% of the vagus nerve will go up into the brain to transmit messages.

Generally, the five internal motor fibers originate from the dorsal nucleus of the vagus nerve of the medulla, and the parasympathetic preganglionic nerve fibers emitted by the nucleus are distributed in the parasympathetic ganglia in or near the organ, and the parasympathetic postganglionic nerve fibers are distributed to the chest.

The organs of the abdominal cavity control the activities of smooth muscle, heart muscle and glands. Generally, the cell body of the five inner sensory fibers is located in the lower ganglion below the jugular foramen, and the central protrusion is stopped in the solitary nucleus, and the pericytes are also distributed in the organs of the chest and the abdomen.

The number of somatosensory fibers is the smallest, and the cell body is located in the upper ganglion of the jugular foramen. The central end of the nucleus is located in the nucleus of the trigeminal nucleus, and the pericytes are distributed in the dura mater and the skin of the auricle and the external auditory canal.

Branches of vagnus nerve

In thyroid surgery, it is possible to accidentally damage the extra larynx lateral branch and recurrent laryngeal nerve. After the injury of the extra cranial nerve branch, the tone is reduced. In the case of recurrent laryngeal nerve injury, due to most of the laryngeal spasm, it may cause hoarseness or difficulty in pronunciation. In bilateral injuries, such as a glottic closure, can cause difficulty breathing and even suffocation.

CRANIAL NERVES

The lower part of our brain is composed of a complex network of nerves that we know as "cranial nerves" or "cranial nerves". In total there are 12, they originate directly in our brain and are distributed along different fibers by means of holes that are at the base of the skull towards the neck, the thorax and the abdomen.

Each of these nerves is composed of fibers that fulfill different functions and that arise from a specific part of the brain (it can be in the base or in the stem).

In turn, each of them has different names according to their origin, their activity, or the specific function they fulfill. In the following sections we will see how it is defined and what functions the vagus nerve has.

Most important branches

Atrial branch (arnold's nerve)

This is one of the four nerve branches that form the superficial cervical plexus. It detaches from the second cervical loop, contours the posterior edge of the sternocleidomastoid and ascends almost vertically towards the atrial pavilion behind the external jugular. Near the angle of the jaw is divided into two branches, one anterior and one posterior.

The anterior branch is distributed through the skin of the outer face of the pavilion and the parotid region. Inside the parotid, you can do anastomosis with the facial. The posterior branch, or atrio-mastoid, is branched by the skin of the internal face of the pavilion and the mastoid region and at this level it can be anastomosed with the mastoid branch that also belongs to the superficial cervical plexus.

Pharyngeal branch

The pterygoid arteries (Vidian arteries) are arteries that reach the ear canal and surrounding area through the pterygoid and form the pharyngeal branch.

It usually originates from the external carotid artery but originates from the internal or external carotid artery or functions as an anastomosis between the two.

From the external carotid artery: The artery passes posteriorly along the pterygoid muscle channel along with the nerves of the pterygoid channel. It is distributed to the upper pharynx and the auditory canal, sending small branches into the tympanic cavity and anastomosing with other tympanic arteries.

From the internal carotid artery: the artery passes posteriorly along the nerves in the pterygoid channel and the pterygoid channel. It is a small, constant branch where the artery leads to the pterygoid canal and anastomoses with the wing ostium branch of the maxillary artery.

Superior laryngeal

Upper laryngeal nerve neuralgia is a rare condition and, therefore, poorly defined clinically in the literature. However, it has precise clinical characteristics and a specific treatment. It has been included in the classification of the International Headache Society and specific diagnostic criteria have been proposed for its detection.

Cardiac branches

In healthy individuals, the electrical activity of the heart is initiated at the sinus node (located at the junction between the superior vena cava and the right atrium). The depolarization wave then propagates to the atrioventricular node (located at the lower part of the right atrium) and then to the cardiac ventricles via the His bundle.

The bundle then divides into two branches, one for each ventricle.

Due to the larger size of the left ventricle, the left branch divides itself in two: one anterior branch and a posterior branch.

The function of these division branches of the His bundle is to drive the electrical pulses and to distribute them in such a way that the contraction of the cardiac muscle is efficient and coordinated.

When a branch is injured, for example during a myocardial infarction or underlying heart disease, it may stop working normally.

This leads to a change in the conduction of cardiac electrical activity: the electrical impulse can no longer spread along the injured limb, it will do through myocardial fibers, a new path that not only slows electrical impulses but change their direction.

As a result, the ability of the ventricles to efficiently pump blood is deteriorated and the amount of blood ejected by the ventricles is reduced.

Cervical branches

The minor occipital nerve or mastoid nerve, with an ascending course, which is distributed to the skin of the mastoid region.

The atrial nerve, ascending, which reaches the skin of the auricular pavilion.

The cutaneous nerve of the neck, of transverse course, and destined to the skin of the supra and sub hyoid region.

The supraclavicular nerve, descending, that innervates the skin of the super lateral part of the thorax.

The supra acromial nerve, which innervates the skin of the shoulder stump

Esophageal plexus branches

The Oesophageal Branches (rami æsophagei) are given off both above and below the bronchial branches; the lower are numerous and larger than the upper. They form, together with the branches of the opposite nerve, the oesophageal plexus. From this plexus filaments are distributed to the back of the pericardium.

Branches of the pulmonary plexus

- Lower cervical branch
- Recurrent laryngeal
- Cardio branches - thoracic
- Anterior vagal trunk
- Posterior vagal trunk

Symptoms of vagus nerve compression

Depending on the importance and type of atlas displacement with respect to its ideal location, pressure on the vagus nerve and / or other cranial nerves, and therefore stimulation, can occur.

If the function of the vagus nerve is impaired (it can also be impaired by cervical osteoarthritis), several symptoms can be verified.

- General sickness
- Heartburn

- Vertigo, dizziness
- Redness of the face
- Tachycardia (rapid heart rate)
- Shoulder stiffness
- Cervical pain
- Headache
- Meniere syndrome
- Difficulty swallowing
- "throat lump"
- Excessive sweating
- Insomnia
- Cold hands or feet
- Irregular or fast heartbeat
- Chronic constipation
- Diarrhea
- Thyroid problems
- Numbness or scalp on one side

Epilepsy is another collateral disease of the vagus nerve. Atlas readjustment is effective for epilepsy.

The traditional medical approach in severe epilepsy episodes is to surgically intervene in the left vagus nerve with a stimulator that is explicitly implanted in the body and cut or inhibit it with an electrical impulse.

Vagus diseases

These diseases generally refer to various types of stimuli that are reflected by the vagus nerve, causing a sudden expansion of the visceral blood vessels and a slowing of the heartbeat, which in turn causes a decrease in blood pressure, hypoxia in the brain, and possibly even a short coma.

A vagus disorder is usually caused by sultry heat and can also occur when fatigue is excessive. At the same time, stress, extreme excitement and anxiety are also the cause of fainting.

THE GENETIC DISEASE OF VERGUS NERVE

It is called Vagotonism. This is a genetic disease of vagus nerve. The HEART depends on emotions and relaxed states. They are two systems,

The SIMPATICO who accelerates him and makes him work quickly and forcefully in case of danger, rage, sexual situations, bad news, also with some drugs, etc.

VAGO is stimulated with calmness, certain drugs, pleasure, moments of rest and sleep, etc. Its action decreases the heart rate, when the heart beats more slowly there is talk of vagotonism. Normal heart rate is 60 to 80. Less than 50 beats per minute is considered Vagotonism, which can lead to death in sleep from a severed slow hear rhythm.

How To Know That The Vagus Nerve Needs To Be Tuned

It is very beneficial to pay attention to the vagus nerve if you feel any of the following sensations:

- Rare sense of taste
- Difficulty swallowing
- Digestion abnormalities
- Sudden changes in heart rate
- Food tasting is difficult
- Facial muscle tension
- Feeling that you cannot speak properly when stressed
- Sudden onset of nausea
- Difficulty in connecting with others
- Excessive negative mental outlook
- Social difficulties

- Tinnitus.

How The "Magical" Vagus Nerve Helps Our Body To Calm Down

The vagus nerve is like the button for our stable emotions. The chief commander of the parasympathetic nervous system

When we face the pressure, the body has to fight or escape, and the vagus nerve plays an important role.

This is why stimulating our vagus nerve can directly affect mood;

This has also proven to be a new technology for the treatment of depression.

Vagal nerve stimulation can also relieve migraine and quickly suppress inflammation.

Our nerves are like the main control buttons that the body restarts.

The word "Vagus" in the vagus nerve refers to the meaning of sputum in Latin. This group of nerves is very long, from the brain to the important organs of the chest and abdomen.

The vagus nerve affects our heartbeat, respiratory system and digestive system. This nerve also transmits information from various organs to the brain. In fact, the (80%) message transmitted by the vagus nerve is almost transmitted from the body to the brain.

This is why the vagus nerve is important to influence our emotions. It monitors whether the organs are functioning well. If the organs of the body work well, the mind is relieved and in a state of satisfaction.

Heart rate variability analysis is an indicator of whether the vagal nerve condition is good. When the vagus nerve tension is large, the heartbeat frequency will decrease slightly during breathing, which is a good phenomenon;

Nerve tension (which also means higher heart rate variability) is strongly correlated with overall health status. Good physical condition includes good digestive system, decreased inflammatory index, strong emotional resilience and longevity;

Low tension is associated with negative emotions, infection, inflammation and heart disease.

People with greater vagal tone will release more oxytocin, and they will have more "altruism"

Active vagus nerves can make people warm and cheerful, and feel the qualities of human nature.

Originally it was thought that the strength of the nerves was static, but now we know that the tension of the vagus nerve can be improved.

How to start your vagus nerve stimulation:

- Take a deep breath (try 4-7-8 tips)
- Yoga
- Meditation
- Spend more time in contact with nature (grounding training)
- Think positively with others

Cultivate healthy intestinal bacteria (because these intestinal probiotics activate the vagus nerve, initiate and release the neurotransmitter gamma-sanobutyric acid in the brain and calm th

Lack of social interaction

Positive social interactions have been shown to cause the activation of the vagus nerve, which means you need that interaction with other people. Even introverts can benefit from talking to someone else, sharing a meal, or engaging in activity that is shared with another person, or multiple people. However, these interactions must remain positive since negative interactions and relationships can actually lower vagus tone.

When interacting with someone else, there are a few ways to increase the vagal tone benefits for both of you. First, establish a meaningful, connected relationship with the other person. This will help both of you. Making eye contact and physical connection can also be beneficial. Hugs are a terrific way to stimulate the vagus nerve, thanks to both physical pressure and positive associations.

You've probably noticed that when you get a hug from someone, it just feels really good. Some people are better huggers than others, but the connection strengthens with hugs and physical contact, making it more likely that you'll continue the relationship and view it in a positive light. All of this is good for your vagal tone and should be pursued whenever possible. It really is this simple.

Chapter 2: The Science of the Vagus Nerve

The vagus nerve is the 10th pair of cranial nerves. It is the longest and most widely distributed pair of cranial nerves, containing sensory, motor and parasympathetic nerve fibers.

The Latin word vagus-of vagor (wandering about, wandering) has an etymological sense-relatedness to the German word. The vagus nerve is usually translated literally as "the wandering nerve". But it could also be translated as "the walking nerve".

Strictly speaking, we speak of two nerve strains, as the vagus nerve is paired, as are many other nerves and organs. That is, they occur twice in the body, one on each side.

The two vagus nerves are rooted in the marrow and originate from the brain base in the area of their transition to the spinal cord. They do this together with other cranial nerves, which do their special services for the human senses.

There are specific nerves, for example, for the balance, the smelling and tasting, the perception and facial expression, perceptions of the larynx, as well as, of course, hearing and sight and others. And these nerves also include the vagus nerve.

After leaving the brain, which, strictly speaking, could be described as a fine protuberance that continues to branch, it nestles with the blood vessels of the cervix, where it also gives off branches to the larynx and other structures, around its long muscles in the direction of the anterior neck lobe, which represents the opening to the chest cavity.

There he begins to branch out more strongly, like the branches of a deciduous tree, which nestle like velvety, holding hands and sensitive fingers around the organs. Heart, lungs, liver, gallbladder, colon, kidneys, bladder, sexual organs, spleen, pancreas, small intestine, stomach, Countless fine branches penetrate into the respective organ tissue and end in depth.

His purely anatomical view conveys something protective, perceptive, sensitive, harmonizing, connecting, a kind of powerful female presence, which conveys comfort and well-being.

The role of the vagus nerve

The vagus nerve dominates breathing, digesting most of the organs of systems, as well as the heart's sensation, movement, and glandular secretion. Therefore, vagal nerve injury can cause circulatory, digestive, and respiratory dysfunction.

The vagus nerve (n. vagus) is a mixed nerve containing four fiber components. Special visceral motor fibers originate from the nucleus of the medulla oblongata, which governs the striated muscles of the pharynx and throat.

Usually visceral motor fibers contribute to the medulla of the dorsal vagal nucleus, which starts at the parasympathetic preganglionic nerve fibers in the organ or near parasympathetic ganglia in the changer neurons after starting parasympathetic postganglionic nerve fibers to the chest, abdomen. These are organs that control the activity of smooth muscle, heart muscle and glands.

The cell body of the visceral sensory fiber is located in the inferior ganglion below the jugular foramen, wherein the central process terminates in the solitary tract nucleus, and the peripheral processes are also distributed in the organs of the chest and abdominal cavity.

Generally, the number of somatosensory fibers is the smallest, and the cell body is located in the upper ganglion of the jugular foramen. The central end of the nucleus is located in the nucleus of the trigeminal nucleus, and the peripheral processes are distributed in the dura mater and the skin of the auricle and the external auditory canal.

Origin of vagus nerve

Its apparent origin is between the accessory cranial nerves (XI) and glossopharyngeal (IX), in the posterior collateral groove of the spinal bulb or retroolivar groove.

Its real origin is found in the cells of the petrosal ganglion, which end at the level of the solitary tract of the bulb.

Our vagus nervous system consists of two opposing systems that always send information to our minds.

The sympathetic nervous system takes adrenaline and cortisol and is part of the fight or flight response, prepare for action and stimulates adrenal glands and sweating.

The parasympathetic nervous system regulates resting internal organs, digestion, and what happens when the body calms down. These two systems bring a tug of war to our hearts, so it is directed to sink the foot into the accelerator. (repetition)

The parasympathetic nervous system is the opposite pole. It is intended to reduce speed, and uses a neurotransmitter such as acetylcholine to reduce heart rate and blood pressure, and to reduce the speed of the heart and organs.

Where the vagus nerve is located

Here's what we are experiencing every day: after eating, we feel tired or a slight drowsiness.

This sensation is regulated by the vagus nerve. After eating, our bodies consume a lot of energy to do digestion.

Therefore, this nerve triggers a series of stimuli to promote calmness and classic "sleepiness".

In addition to controlling digestion, the vagus nerve monitors that the heart is not overexcited. Therefore, the vagus nerve causes loss of consciousness if something is seriously wrong.

It also regulates the immune system and cell regeneration. On the other hand, another feature of this attractive structure is to give you a feeling of fullness.

Since it is closely related to the digestive process, it also functions as a regulator.

This tells us that we already have enough, and when we suffer from stress, it tells us that we have more cravings or less appetite.

As you can see, it is a natural complement in various fields, such as relaxation, fullness, weight, and more or less anxiety.

Vagus nerve path

Vagus nerve is the longest stroke in the brain, the most widely distributed nerve at glossopharyngeal nerve filaments under the brain via the jugular foramen the cranial cavity.

Then, it descends to the back of the neck, between the common carotid artery and the internal jugular vein, and enters the thoracic cavity through the thoracic upper mouth. In the chest, the left and right vagus nerves travel in different positions

Its path begins in the cells of the petrosal ganglion, then goes through the jugular hole (posterior tear) of the skull base and reaches the retro-stellar space.

In this space, it joins the internal carotid artery and the internal jugular vein, forming with them the main neck veins.

Thus, it descends through the neck encompassed in this package.

In its descent it emits the superior laryngeal nerve, and also gives branches for the pharynx.

Once inside the thorax, the right and left vagus nerves behave differently:

LEFT VAGUS NERVE

It enters the thorax between the left carotid and left subclavian arteries, and at the height of the aortic arch it emits the left recurrent laryngeal nerve.

Then it goes down and forward (becomes anterior) and passes behind the pulmonary pedicle before reaching the esophagus, where it contributes to form the esophageal plexus.

RIGHT VAGUS NERVE

It crosses in front of the right subclavian artery, and at this height it emits the right recurrent laryngeal nerve.

Then it goes down and back (it becomes posterior) and passes behind the right pulmonary pedicle before reaching the esophagus, where it also helps to form the esophageal plexus, just like its left counterpart.

Within the thorax, the vagus nerves give branches to the cardiac plexus and the pulmonary plexus.

Both vagus nerves make the last part of their journey through the thorax along with the esophagus, and next to it the abdominal cavity is introduced, crossing the diaphragm through the esophageal hiatus.

Once in the abdominal cavity, the left vagus nerve is distributed through the stomach, while the right vagus nerve ends in the solar plexus from where it gives branches for the abdominal viscera (stomach, intestines, kidneys and liver).

IT IS CONSIDERED A MIXED NERVE WITH DIFFERENT REFERENCES

Vasovagal SYNCOPE

This is a common form of fainting. Various situations can stimulate the vagus nerve, which causes a reduction in heart rate and a dilation of the body's blood vessels through the parasympathetic system. The heart rate slows and dilated blood vessels cause less blood to reach the brain, thus causing fainting.

Vasovagal syncope is reflex type. There are situational syncopes that occur at times such as urinating, defecating, swallowing or coughing. The causes of syncope have not been fully understood but it is believed that they occur in people with excessive peripheral venous load, resulting in a sudden drop in peripheral venous return.

This results in a state of cardiac hyper-contractility that activates the responsive mechanoreceptors to stretch thus limiting the conditions of hypotension and causes a decrease in heart rate below 60 beats per minute (normal is 60 to 80 beats per minute).

TRIGGERS

The triggers of vasovagal syncope are those that produce an increase in parasympathetic activity in sensitive people. The main ones, although not the only ones:

Drastic changes of position (when getting up very fast, yoga, Pilates, doing abdominal exercises, etc.)

- Standing for a long time
- Sitting for a long time
- Emotional stress
- Any pain
- Non-pleasant stimulations such as:
- Donate blood
- Prolonged exposure to heat
- Extreme emotions

- Hunger

- Anxiety

- Conglomeration of people

- Nausea or vomiting

- Dehydration

- Difficult Urination or defecation

- Swallowing

- Hard severe coughing

- Colic

- Altitude change

- Pressure in certain places of the throat, nose and eyes

- Venous punctures

- Dental surgery

- Unpleasant odors

- Chemical odors (paint, chlorine, resistol, etc.)

- Use of diuretics

- Restriction of salt in the diet

- Alcohol intake or a very copious meal

- Do strong exercises in a very hot climate

- Drug use, alcohol

- Allergy to medications.

- Amusement park rides

CLINICAL CHARACTERISTICS

Most syncopes (75%) in patients with a "healthy heart" are due to vasovagal syncope. Approximately 70% of patients are under sixty-five years old, being more frequent in women than in men. These patients have a high incidence of neuropsychiatric disorders and some suffer from psychogenic syncope.

Although some of these patients may present orthostatic hypotension to a greater or lesser degree, most have normal blood pressure between syncopal episodes. In many cases the syncope is preceded by prodromes (which can last from seconds to minutes), among them we have:

- Yawns
- Epigastric discomfort
- Weakness
- Paresthesia
- Hot
- Anxiety
- Visual field decline
- Hyperventilation
- Palpitations
- Pallor
- Diaphoresis
- Sickness
- Dizziness
- Vertigo
- Feeling that the ears are covered
- Gradual ringing in the ears.

- Shortness of breath or walking

- Feeling of imminent fainting

Prodromes do not always occur resulting in sudden loss of consciousness, so the risk of physical injuries from actually falling are greater. These atypical situations, without prodromes, are more frequent in the elderly.

While the typical form, initially described, is more common in younger patients, usually teenagers. It occurs in young adults with the same consequences, and it is the least researched disease in the English-speaking world so many doctors determine that we should only get used to it without taking medication, and that worsens the quality of life in many cases.

During the syncopal episode you may have one or more of the following symptoms:

- Pallor
- Profuse sweating
- Cold skin
- Dilated pupils
- Fainting without fainting
- Mental confusion and lack of guidance
- And less frequently fecal or urinary incontinence.

Also in some cases, tonic or colonic movements can be observed, indicating that the cerebral anoxic threshold was reached (the brain stops receiving oxygen). The loss of consciousness is brief, with a rapid recovery when changing the position of the body.

When crises begin in adolescence, they usually decrease over time. In young women the episodes become more frequent during the menstrual period. In patients with recurrent syncope's, a higher incidence of neuropsychiatric disorders (depressions, somatizations, panic disorders), and neurosomatics, such as vascular problems and functional digestive problems, have been found. It has also been linked to Chronic Fatigue Syndrome.

DIAGNOSTICS

A more than important number of conditions can cause this syncope. Making a correct diagnosis of loss of consciousness is one of the most difficult challenges a doctor can face. The basis of a good diagnosis of vasovagal syncope and other diseases is based on a clear description by the patient, especially on the triggering events, the symptoms and when it occurs.

In patients with recurrence of this syncope, the appropriate diagnosis can be made with one or more of the following medical tests or tests:

- Tilt table test
- Implementation of a "loop" type insert recorder.
- Holter-monitor or some other type of heart monitor
- An echocardiogram
- A study of cardiac electrophysiology
- Try to touch the tip of the nose alternately with the tip of the index fingers of each hand.

TREATMENT

As general measures, the nature of the problem must be explained to the patient and instructed to avoid the predisposing factors (extreme heat, dehydration, conglomerates of people, etc.), as well as to recognize the premonitory symptoms, so that, when presenting these, can adopt a position of decubitus and perform maneuvers that increase venous return.

When there are factors that limit preload, such as inadequate venous return or chronic hypovolemia (e.g., use of diuretics, etc.), it may be that the symptoms disappear by correcting these factors (adjustments in diuretic doses, use of compressive elastic stockings, among others).

It is very important to instruct the patient to increase the intake of salt and fluids in their diet. You can exercise, but you should be instructed to consume hydrating drinks before and after it.

There are two types of treatment for vasovagal syncope, the change in lifestyle being preferable because drugs and devices have side effects that may affect more than they benefit. Each treatment should be individualized in each patient according to the clinical manifestations and the result of the Tilt Test.

LIFESTYLE

Fluid intake of at least two liters a day to stay hydrated.

Salt intake (7 grams per day; approximately 1 1/2 teaspoon)

Physical maneuvers: isometric contraction of arms (there is muscle contraction, which develops tension, but no movement. For example, I remain locked in the bar with folded arms), cross my legs and squeeze

Tilt training: 10 to 30 minutes per day standing against the wall

Lie down and lift your feet on a wall higher than your head for five to ten minutes three times a day.

- Increase daily fluid intake to avoid dehydration
- In case of exercise and profuse sweating or women during menstrual periods ingest hydrating products with electrolytes (Gatorade, etc.)
- Do not restrict salt in the diet
- Avoid extreme heat.

Chapter 3: What Happens When Vagus Nerve Malfunctions

Damage to the vagus nerve can produce a range of symptoms because the nerves are long and affect many areas of the body.

Potential symptoms of vagus nerve damage include: difficulty speaking or losing voice, hoarseness or wheezing, difficulty drinking water, disappearing vomiting reflex, ear pain, abnormal heart rhythms, abnormal blood pressure, decreased production of stomach acid, nausea or vomiting, abdominal distension or pain. The symptoms someone may experience depend on which part of the nerve is damaged.

Gastroparesis

Specialists believe that harm to the vagus nerve may also cause gastroparesis. This condition affects the involuntary contraction of the digestive system and prevents normal gastric emptying. If you have ever had this it is very uncomfortable. Basically it feels like there is a lump in your throat, or the "pill stuck in the esophagus" sensation.

Other symptoms of gastroparesis include nausea or vomiting, especially undigested food vomiting several hours after eating, loss of appetite or fullness shortly after eating, acid reflux, abdominal pain or bloating, unexplained weight loss, and blood sugar fluctuations. Some people develop gastroparesis after vagus nerve amputation surgery, which removes all or part of the vagus nerve.

Vagal syncope-sometimes the vagus nerve overreacts to certain stress triggers, such as exposure to extreme temperatures, severe anxiety, lack of sleep or extreme dehydration. Often gastroparesis develops when someone is not sleeping properly.

Remember also that the vagus nerve stimulates certain muscles in the heart, which can help slow your heart rate. Overreaction can cause a sudden drop in heart rate and blood pressure, which can lead to syncope. This is called vasovagal syncope.

Scientists have long known that chronic diseases such as alcoholism and diabetes can damage nerves, including the vagus nerve, although the scientific cause of this damage is unknown. People with insulin-dependent diabetes may develop neuropathy in many nerves. If the vagus nerve is damaged, it can cause nausea, bloating, diarrhea and gastroparesis (stomach emptying too slowly/lump in throat sensation).

Unfortunately, diabetic neuropathy cannot be reversed. If the vagus nerve is damaged due to trauma or tumor growth, it may cause digestive symptoms or hoarseness, vocal cord paralysis, and slowed heart rate. In a few people with minimal damage to the vagus nerve, nerves can regenerate after tumor removal.

Vagus and syncope: When someone faints due to heat, standing for a long time, or standing up really fast(such as seeing bloodstains), it should be attributed to the vagus nerve. This phenomenon is called vasovagal syncope, which occurs when the sympathetic nerve divides and expands the blood vessels in the legs.

When the vagus nerve overreacts, the heart rate immediately drops significantly. There is a blood pool in the leg, blood pressure drops, and there is not enough blood flowing to the brain, and the person will temporarily lose consciousness. Unless an individual faints frequently, vasovagal syncope does not require any treatment.

How To Diagnose Vagus Nerve Damage

The vagus nerve, which is known as the tenth cranial nerve or X cranial nerve, and the most complex cranial nerve, is responsible for telling the stomach muscles to contract when eating so they can digest the food. When it does not work, it can cause gastroparesis, which is a slower gastric emptying. To determine if the vagus nerve is damaged, pay attention to the symptoms of gastroparesis, and then consult a doctor who may order a diagnostic test for you.

Obviously the biggest symptom of this is when food takes longer to pass through the system. Gastroparesis prevents food from passing through your body at a regular rate. If you're less likely to go to the toilet, it may indicate that you have gastroparesis.

Take note of diarrhea and fatigue. Nausea and vomiting are typical gastroparesis signs. Because there's no emptying of your mouth, the food is lying there, making you uncomfortable. Yes, you will find that the food is not digested at all when you vomit. It is possible that this symptom will happen every day.

Watch for heartburn. Heartburn is also a common symptom of the disease. Heartburn is a chest and throat sensation caused by acid reflux. You may experience this symptom frequently.

Check if your appetite is low. This disease reduces appetite because the food you eat is not properly digested. This means that new food has nowhere to go, so you won't feel hungry. In fact, you may feel full after taking a few bites. This is great for weight loss but not good for nutrition requirements.

Weight Loss. Because you don't want to eat too much, you may lose weight. Also, your stomach doesn't digest food as it should, so you don't get the nutrients you need to fuel your body and maintain your weight.

Look for pain and bloating of the stomach. Because food stays in the stomach longer than it should, you may feel bloating. Again, this situation can make your stomach hurt or just feel plain uncomfortable.

If you are a diabetic, be aware of blood glucose changes. This disease is common in type 1 and type 2 diabetes. If you find that your blood glucose reading is more erratic than normal, it may also be a sign of this problem.

Seek medical attention if multiple symptoms are found. If you notice these signs for more than a week at the same time, make an appointment with a doctor as the disease can cause serious complications. It can cause you to become dehydrated or malnourished because your body cannot get the food it needs through digestion.

List your symptoms. Whenever you see a doctor, it is best to list your symptoms. Write down the symptoms you have always had and when, so your doctor can get a good idea of your condition. It also helps you remember everything you need to do when you go to the hospital. Perform physical and diagnostic tests. The doctor will ask you questions about your medical history and give you a physical examination. They may feel your stomach and use a stethoscope to listen to the area. They may also perform imaging studies to help you identify the cause of the symptoms.

Present any risk factors, including diabetes and abdominal surgery. Other risk factors include hypothyroidism, infections, neurological diseases and scleroderma.

Get a endoscope or X-ray examination. Your doctor may order these tests first to make sure you don't have a blocked stomach. Gastric obstruction can cause symptoms similar to gastroparesis. For endoscopy, your doctor will use a miniature camera on the hose. First, you will get a sedative and you may feel tingling in your throat. The tube will pass through the back of the throat and into the esophagus and upper digestive tract. Compared to using X-rays, the camera will help your doctor understand more directly what is going on. You may also receive a similar test called an esophageal manometry test to measure gastric contractions. In this case, the test tube will be inserted through your nose and left for 15 minutes.

If doctors find no obstructions on other tests, they may order the study. This test is a bit interesting. You will eat something with low radiation and the doctor will then check how long it takes you to digest it with your imager. Usually if half of your food remains in the stomach after an hour to an hour and a half, you will get a diagnosis of gastroparesis. An ultrasound will help your doctor detect if there are other problems that are causing your symptoms. In particular, they will check how well your kidneys and gallbladder are performing in this test.

Prepare for an electrocardiogram. If your doctor has difficulty explaining your symptoms, you may need to complete this test. Basically, this is a way to listen to your stomach for an hour. They will place the electrodes outside your abdomen. You must perform this test on an empty stomach.

Symptoms Of Vagus Nerve Dysfunction

Not many people actually know what a vagus nerve is. The vagus nerve is the lengthiest crane nerve throughout the body. It helps to regulate the intestines and affects the cardiovascular, immune, endocrine and respiratory systems. This means that the nerve in the human body is very important. Whenever that nerve is dysfunctional, you can imagine it produces some very ridiculous side effects.

Interestingly, vagus nerve dysfunction is common with many people. When you are struggling with vagus nerve dysfunction, you can be in a fully healthy state for a long time, catch a cold or hit a wall, and your body will take months to recover.

Vagus insufficiency is something that must be coped with in life, because there is no ultimate immediate cure.

Aggressive behavior, anxiety, anger, sadness, depression, fear, etc. may exist, although in many cases the cause or motivation does not exist. However, in addition to lack of motivation, indifference, reluctance, and difficulty remembering certain events may be the reason behind the above process. If these behaviors do not disappear quickly, measures should be taken to avoid this situation due to the mentioned feedback mechanism. Damage to the vagus nerve as it passes through the throat can cause difficulty speaking and swallowing.

It may also cause digestive problems, loss of appetite or vice versa, no matter how little you eat, we will feel full. If the vagus nerve becomes inflamed, we may experience nausea, heartburn, dizziness, headache, tachycardia, pain and stiff neck, vomiting or the so-called "vagus nerve crisis", whose symptoms are heavy sweating, pale, discomfort and even syncope. The symptoms of damage depend on the severity of the injury, the location, and whether nearby blood vessels are also affected.

Chronic diseases can damage any nerve, including the vagus nerve, so people with diseases such as diabetes should discuss the possibility of neurological complications with their doctor. Once again, the main cause of damage to the vagus nerve is diabetes in any form, even pre-diabetes. Secondary would be alcohol and drug abuse, and thirdly would be poor dietary choices.

Smoking and drinking can exacerbate nerve damage. If any symptoms appear, it is necessary to consult a doctor in order to obtain the correct diagnosis and determine the possible root cause. If the vagus nerve becomes inflamed, its function will be logically affected. It may be caused by the so-called vagus syndrome, which is characterized by nausea, heartburn, dizziness, headache, tachycardia, pain and stiffness in the neck, vomiting or vagus nerve crisis, directly involving the heart and showing some symptoms of discomfort, For example, excessive sweating, pale face, general weakness, nausea and even fainting.

The following are several more symptoms of vagus nerve dysfunction:

1. Chronic nausea

2. Weight loss: Because you don't feel like eating, you can lose weight.

3. Weight gain

4. Bradycardia and tachycardia: called heart rate decrease and heart rate increase, respectively. This can make it difficult for easy things like walking or standing for long periods of time, getting dizzy when standing up, etc.

5. IBS: Persistent stomach pain and nausea usually means constant discomfort.

6. Depression: Not only because it is connected to your brain, but always feeling depressed and uncomfortable will definitely damage your mental health.

7. Anxiety

8. Chronic inflammation

9. Chronic fatigue

10. Heartburn

11. Dizziness / fainting:

12. Voice changes. When the vagus nerve is damaged, the branches of the throat are affected.

13. Difficulty swallowing. The vagus nerve controls many muscles of the upper jaw and tongue, and if damaged, can cause difficulty swallowing (dysphagia).

14. Change in gag reflection. The vagus nerve controls the vomiting reflex, so the injury may cause the reflex to disappear.

15. Loss of hearing.

16. Cardiovascular problems. This can manifest again as rhythm abnormalities.

17. Digestive problems. Damage to the vagus nerve can cause many issues from improper digestion, one being weight gain.

Complications:

<u>Damage to the vagus nerve can cause the stomach muscles stop functioning normally.</u> A healthy stomach contracts, pushing food into the small intestine.

Vagus lesions can interfere with this function, causing food to move slowly or stop passing through the digestive system altogether. Symptoms of gastroparesis include feeling full after eating a small amount of food, losing weight, heartburn and nausea. Drug management and some dietary changes can help resolve the symptoms of gastroparesis.

Vagus nerve dysfunction is usually caused by a low vagal tone index, so stimulation of the vagus nerve can be used as a treatment for signs, symptoms, and disease. Many of these treatments represent lifestyle changes, which means that it is safe to use more than one of the following practices to increase the vagus tone index.

Chapter 4: Common Problems It Can Heal

Vagus nerve incitement includes the utilization of a gadget to animate the vagus nerve with electrical motivations. An implantable vagus nerve trigger is, as of now, FDA-endorsed to treat epilepsy and sadness. There's one vagus nerve on each side of your body, running from your brainstem through your neck to your chest and stomach area.

In ordinary vagus nerve incitement, a gadget is carefully embedded under the skin on your chest, and a wire is strung under your skin, interfacing the gadget to one side vagus nerve. At the point when initiated, the gadget sends an electrical flag along the left vagus nerve to your brainstem, which at that point, sends a sign to specific regions in your mind. The correct vagus nerve isn't utilized in light of the fact that it's bound to convey strands that supply nerves to the heart.

New, noninvasive vagus nerve incitement gadgets, which don't require careful implantation, have been affirmed in Europe to treat epilepsy, sadness, and torment. A noninvasive gadget that animates the vagus nerve was as of late endorsed by the Food and Drug Administration for the treatment of group migraines in the United States.

Around 33% of individuals with epilepsy don't completely react to hostile to seizure drugs. Vagus nerve incitement might be a choice to diminish the recurrence of seizures in individuals who haven't accomplished control with meds.

Vagus nerve incitement may likewise be useful for individuals who haven't reacted to escalated melancholy medicines, for example, energizer prescriptions, mental guiding (psychotherapy), and electroconvulsive treatment (ECT).

The Food and Drug Administration (FDA) has endorsed vagus nerve incitement for individuals who:

- Have central (incomplete) epilepsy
- Have seizures that aren't well-controlled with meds

The FDA has likewise endorsed vagus nerve incitement for the treatment of depression in adults who:

1. Have ceaseless, difficult-to-treat melancholy (treatment-safe despondency)
2. Haven't improved in the wake of attempting at least four prescriptions or electroconvulsive treatment (ECT), or both
3. Proceed with standard sorrow medicines alongside vagus nerve incitement

Moreover, specialists are examining vagus nerve incitement as a potential treatment for an assortment of conditions, including cerebral pains, rheumatoid joint inflammation, provocative entrail infection, bipolar issue, heftiness, and Alzheimer's ailment.

Dangers

For a great many people, vagus nerve incitement is protected. In any case, it has a few dangers, both from the medical procedure to embed the gadget and from the mind incitement.

Medical procedure dangers

Careful complexities with embedded vagus nerve incitement are uncommon and are like the threats of having different kinds of medical procedures. They include:

- Torment where the (cut) is made to embed the gadget

- Disease

- Trouble gulping

- Vocal rope loss of motion, which is normally transitory, yet can be lasting

- Reactions after a medical procedure

A portion of the reactions and medical issues related to embedded vagus nerve incitement can include:

- Voice changes

- Hoarse voice

- Throat torment

- Hacking cough

- Cerebral pains

- Shortness of breath

- Trouble swallowing

- Shivering or prickling of the skin

- Sleeping disorders

- Declining of rest apnea

For the vast majority, reactions are passable. They may reduce after some time, yet some symptoms may stay irksome for whatever length of time that you utilize embedded vagus nerve incitement.

Changing the electrical driving forces can help limit these impacts. In the event that symptoms are unfortunate, the gadget can be closed off briefly or for all time.

How to plan

It's imperative to deliberately consider the upsides and downsides of embedded vagus nerve incitement before choosing to have the technique. Ensure you realize what the entirety of your other treatment decisions are and that you and your primary care physician both feel that embedded vagus nerve incitement is the best choice for you. Ask your primary care physician precisely what you ought to expect during a medical procedure and after they beat generator is set up.

Nourishment and drugs

You may need to quit taking certain drugs early, and your PCP may ask you not to eat the night prior to the system.

What you can anticipate

Prior to the methodology

Prior to a medical procedure, your PCP will do a physical assessment. You may require blood tests or different tests to ensure you don't have any wellbeing worries that may be an issue. Your primary care physician may have you start taking anti-microbials before medical procedures to avoid disease.

During the technique

Medical procedure to embed the vagus nerve incitement gadget should be possible on an outpatient premise. However, a few specialists suggest remaining medium-term.

The medical procedure, for the most part, takes an hour to 90 minutes. You may stay conscious yet have drugs to numb the medical procedure territory (nearby anesthesia), or you might be oblivious during the medical procedure (general anesthesia).

Two cuts are made, one on your chest or in the armpit (axillary) district, and the other on the left half of the neck.

The electrical generator is embedded in the upper left half of your chest. The gadget is intended to be a perpetual embed. However, it tends to be expelled if important.

The beat generator is about the size of a stopwatch and runs on battery control. A lead wire is associated with the heartbeat generator. The lead wire is guided under your skin from your chest up to your neck, where it's appended to one side vagus nerve during that time entry point.

After the methodology

The beat generator is turned on during a visit to your primary care physician's office half a month after a medical procedure. At that point, it very well may be customized to convey electrical motivations to the vagus nerve at different terms, frequencies, and flows. Vagus nerve incitement, for the most part, begins at a low level and is slowly expanded, contingent upon your indications and reactions.

Incitement is customized to turn on and off in explicit cycles —, for example, 30 seconds on, five minutes off. You may have shiver sensations or slight annoyance when the nerve incitement is on.

The trigger doesn't recognize seizure action or melancholy side effects. At the point when it's turned on, the trigger turns on and off at the interims chose by your PCP. You can utilize a hand-held magnet to start incitement at an alternate time, for instance, in the event that you sense a looming seizure.

The magnet can likewise be utilized to incidentally kill the vagus nerve incitement, which might be essential when you do certain exercises, for example, open talking, singing, or working out, or when you're eating in the event that you have swallowing issues.

You'll have to visit your primary care physician occasionally to ensure that the beat generator is working accurately and that it hasn't moved out of position. Check with your primary care physician before having any restorative tests, for example, attractive reverberation imaging (MRI), which may meddle with your gadget.

Results

Embedded vagus nerve incitement isn't a solution for epilepsy. A great many people with epilepsy won't quit having seizures or taking epilepsy medicine inside and out after the methodology. However, many will have fewer seizures, up to 20 to 50 percent less. Seizure force may diminish too.

It can take months or even a year or longer of incitement before you see any critical decrease in seizures. Vagus nerve incitement may likewise abbreviate the recuperation time after a seizure. Individuals who've had vagus nerve incitement to treat epilepsy may likewise encounter upgrades in disposition and personal satisfaction.

Research is as yet undecided on the advantages of embedded vagus nerve incitement for the treatment of discouragement. A few investigations recommend the advantages of vagus nerve incitement for discouragement gather after some time, and it might take at any rate a while of treatment before you see any enhancements in your downturn side effects. Embedded vagus nerve incitement doesn't work for everyone, and it isn't proposed to supplant conventional medicines.

Fiery reactions assume a focal job in the advancement and determination of numerous ailments and can prompt incapacitating ceaseless torment. As a rule, aggravation is your body's reaction. In this way, decreasing "battle or-flight" reactions in the sensory system and bringing down organic markers for stress can likewise diminish irritation.

Ordinarily, specialists endorse prescriptions to battle irritation. Nonetheless, there's developing proof that another method to battle irritation is by connecting with the vagus nerve and improving "vagal tone." This can be accomplished through every day activities, for example, yoga and contemplation—or in progressively outrageous instances of aggravation, for example, rheumatoid joint inflammation (RA)— by utilizing an embedded gadget for vagus nerve incitement (VNS).

The vagus nerve is known as the "meandering nerve" since it has different branches that veer from two thick stems established in the cerebellum and brainstem that meander to the least viscera of your belly contacting your heart and most significant organs en route. Vagus signifies "meandering" in Latin. The words drifter, ambiguous, and transient are altogether gotten from a similar Latin root.

In 1921, a German physiologist named Otto Loewi found that animating the vagus nerve caused a decrease in pulse by setting off the arrival of a substance he instituted Vagusstoff (German for "Vagus Substance"). The "vagus substance" was later distinguished as acetylcholine and turned into the primary synapse at any point recognized by researchers.

Vagusstoff (acetylcholine) resembles a sedative that you can self-direct essentially by taking a couple of full breaths with long breathes out. Deliberately taking advantage of the intensity of your vagus nerve can make a condition of internal quiet while subduing your irritation reflex.

The vagus nerve is the prime segment of the parasympathetic sensory system, which directs the "rest-and-digest" or "tend-and-get to know" reactions. On the other side, to look after homeostasis, the thoughtful sensory system drives the "battle or flight" reaction.

Sound vagal tone is shown by a slight increment of the pulse when you breathe in, and a reduction of the pulse when you breathe out. Profound diaphragmatic breathing — with a long, slow breathe out — is vital to invigorating the vagus nerve and easing back pulse and circulatory strain, particularly in the midst of execution nervousness.

A higher vagal tone record is connected to physical and mental prosperity. Alternately, a low vagal tone list is related to aggravation, sadness, negative states of mind, forlornness, coronary failures, and stroke.

A recent report, "How Positive Emotions Build Physical Health: Perceived Positive Social Connections Account for the Upward Spiral Between Positive Emotions and Vagal Tone," was distributed in Psychological Science. For this examination, Barbara Fredrickson and Bethany Kok of the University of North Carolina at Chapel Hill focused on the vagus nerve and found that a high vagal tone record was a piece of a criticism circle between positive feelings, physical wellbeing, and positive social associations.

Their examination proposes that positive feelings, powerful social associations, and physical wellbeing impact each other in a self-supporting upward winding dynamic and input circle that researchers are simply starting to comprehend.

For this examination, Frederickson and Kok utilized a Loving-Kindness Meditation (LKM) method to assist members with getting better at self-producing positive feelings. In any case, they additionally found that essentially considering positive social associations and attempting to improve affectionate human bonds likewise caused enhancements in vagal tone.

In 2014, I composed a Psychology Today blog entry, "How Does the Vagus Nerve Convey Gut Instincts to the Brain?" in view of discoveries by specialists in Switzerland who recognized how the vagus nerve passes on "premonitions" of nervousness and dread to the mind. Clinical and trial contemplates showing that pressure and melancholy are related with the up-guideline of the resistant framework, including expanded generation of expert fiery cytokines.

When directed to patients or research facility creatures, cytokines have been found to incite regular side effects of misery. Along these lines, a few instances of a low state of mind, low vitality, and absence of inspiration might be because of raised degrees of cytokine proteins.

Vagus Nerve Stimulation (VNS) Dramatically Reduces Arthritic Inflammation

As of late, a global group of specialists from Amsterdam and the United States led a clinical preliminary which exhibits that invigorating the vagus nerve with a little embedded gadget essentially decreased aggravation and improved results for patients with rheumatoid joint pain by repressing cytokine generation.

RA is a constant provocative ailment that influences roughly 1.3 million individuals in the United States and costs several billions of dollars to treat every year, as per the analysts.

The neuroscientists and immunology specialists engaged with this examination utilized best in class innovation to delineate neural hardware that manages irritation. In one circuit — named "the incendiary reflex" — activity possibilities transmitted in the vagus nerve repress the generation of provocative professional cytokines.

The July 2016 investigation, "*Vagus Nerve Stimulation Inhibits Cytokine Production and Attenuates Disease Severity in Rheumatoid Arthritis,*" is online in the Proceedings of the National Academy of Sciences (PNAS) and will be distributed in a future coming print issue.

This investigation intended to decrease side effects of rheumatoid joint pain by invigorating the vagus nerve with a little embedded gadget, subsequently set off a chain response that diminished cytokine levels and irritation. In spite of the fact that this investigation concentrated on rheumatoid joint pain, the preliminary's outcomes may have suggestions for patients experiencing other provocative infections, including Parkinson's, Crohn's, and Alzheimer's.

In an announcement, Paul-Peter Tak, the global head specialist and lead creator of the paper from the Division of Clinical Immunology and Rheumatology of the Academic Medical Center at the University of Amsterdam, stated,

"This is the primary investigation to assess in the case of animating the provocative reflex straightforwardly with an embedded electronic gadget can treat RA in people. We have recently demonstrated that focusing on the incendiary reflex may decrease aggravation in creature models and in vitro models of RA . . . which may be pertinent for other insusceptible interceded incendiary infections too."

These discoveries propose another way to deal with battling infections that are at present treated with moderately costly medications that have a large group of symptoms. VNS gives medicinal services suppliers a possibly increasingly viable approach to improve the lives of individuals experiencing ceaseless provocative ailments.

How Improving The Vagal Tone Can Prevent Physical Inflammation

Inflammation is often just a battle between your body and contaminations, but it is widespread today, adding to various sicknesses, including sepsis. In spite of the fact that sepsis is regularly caused by a disease, serious sepsis kills more than 250,000 Americans consistently, notwithstanding the viability of the new anti-toxins.

Epidemiological examinations show that physical exercise is among the most significant elements controlling the resistant framework and improving personal satisfaction. Exercise diminishes the danger of numerous conditions, including cardiovascular ailments, hypertension, atherosclerosis, metabolic disorder, diabetes, joint pain, pneumonic issue, dementia, and many other kinds of diseases. Long term exercise prevents metabolic issues, yet it's anything but an achievable choice for patients with bad habits or constrained versatility.

Serious anaerobic exercise instigates metabolic pressure, including hypoglycemia, while long term aerobic incites physiological adjustment improving resting pulse, respiratory sinus arrhythmia and cardiovascular vagal tone. Long term aerobic exercise seems to be the much better choice.

Customary exercise decreases instinctive fat mass. Accordingly, aerobic preparing can likewise counteract aggravation by diminishing the creation of adipokines, provocative variables delivered by adipocytes and fat tissue. In like manner, customary exercising likewise initiates alterations in resistant and non-insusceptible tissue, decreasing the generation of provocative factors macrophages.

There is an old Chinese cure that helps invigorate the vagus nerve. Generally, what's known as a "hot and cold dive" where you sit in heated water then place your face in ice water for 20 seconds and rehashing it 5-10 times additionally are exceptionally effective in vagal incitement, as outlined earlier in this book.

Gut issues.

The enteric sensory system — or what is portrayed now and then as the gut's sensory system — interfaces with the mind through the vagus nerve. There is expanding proof indicating an impact of the gut microbiota on the mind. People enhanced with L. rhamnosus experienced different positive changes in GABA receptors that were intervened by the vagus nerve.

Eating the right foods and taking probiotics to keep your gut biology steady and sound. Additionally, irregular fasting or lessening calories has appeared to be a marker of vagal tone.

Lessen jaw pressure.

The jaw is identified with both the trigeminal and vagus nerve, and the misalignment of the jaw can cause a low vagal tone.

On the off chance that you have had implanted supports, extensive oral work, or have insecure hips and poor foot quality, you are at higher risk for low vagal tone.

All things considered, there are treatments for those with the low vagal tone, and the jaw can be a quick solution. One is the thing that we call the fast in and out facelift. It's initially built up for those with jaw torment. You can do it anyplace, and it works quickly. By animating the tissue where the vagus nerve fans out behind the ears, you can diminish the pressure the tissue regularly has at the base of the skull. This is regularly a guilty party to vagal issues missed in treatment. Now and again, the nerve is, in reality, fine, yet the tissue encompassing it makes lopsided electrical misfires in its association with mind-gut. By discharging the tissues here with either this method or the neck discharge grouping, you can rapidly help the equalization and association the vagus nerve needs to work productively.

Decompress your neck. The Neck Release Sequence can without much of a stretch reduce tension in your body, diminish pointless joint pressure, and immediately impact vagal tone. Discharging neck pressure with this straightforward succession additionally lessens strains or tensions in the chest area where the nerve stretches out at the neck space.

Dissolve your hands and feet. Treat your hands and feet to a MELT treatment as regularly as consistently to reenact the liquid stream all through the whole connective tissue framework just as the billions of tangible nerve endings found in your hands and feet. The areas on the back of the hands and feet all identify with our organs. So this is an aberrant method to enable the autonomic sensory system to reestablish entire body balance in as little as 10 minutes every day.

Chapter 5: P.T.S.D.

Post-traumatic stress disorder is an anxiety disorder that can improve after trauma and is characterized by experiencing intrusive memories, flashbacks, hypervigilance, nightmares, social avoidance and social dilemmas. The signs of PTSD can be classified into four groups: intrusive symptoms, avoidance behavior, cognitive and affective changes and deficiency in sexual arousal and response. People undergoing PTSD have a will to live, although under an everlasting danger. They show combat and fight behavior against continuous behavior closure and segregation with no opportunity to achieve a calm state of mind and develop wonderful social relationships. Over time, these disordered autonomic reactions lead to the development of an extended threat to psychiatric comorbidities, such as addiction and cardiovascular diseases.

Post traumatic stress disorder signals are transmitted partly through the vagus nerve. There is evidence for a reduced parasympathetic activity in PTSD sufferers, indicating an autonomic imbalance.

Vagal manipulation of the coronary arteries through myelinated vagal fibers varies with that of the respiratory organs. Thus, the effect on the respiratory sinus arrhythmia(RSA) can be assessed by measuring the amplitude of rhythmic fluctuations in heart rate. A recent finding has shown that reducing RSA in veterans with PTSD provides comfort. In addition, patients with PTSD have been shown to have less high-frequency heart rate variability.

The continued change of emotional cues to conditioned cues is one of several hallmarks of PTSD despite the absence of additional trauma. The behavior employed to deal with PTSD depends on the affected person supporting the affected person to reduce his or her anxiety about this cue over time. Thus, exposure-based treatment plans are considered to be the preferred therapy for PTSD. The intention of exposure-based therapies is to replace conditional associations of trauma with new, more deviant associations that compete with fearful associations. Studies have proven that fear of extinction in patients with PTSD, as well as activation of the fear extinction system, is also missed. This system includes the ventromedial prefrontal cortex, the amygdala and the hippocampus. This is not particularly necessary for the contextual retrieval of anxiety memories after extinction.

Post traumatic stress disorder shows severe structural abnormalities related to the anterior hippocampus, ventromedial prefrontal cortex and amygdala. There is evidence of activation of the amygdala in humans and rodents for a period of conditioned fear. The amygdala and the PFC have reciprocal synaptic connections. In fact, due to uncertainty and danger, the PFC may become hypoactive due to failure to inhibit the overgrowth of the amygdala with the emergence of PTSD symptoms and even re-experiencing it.

The hippocampus is additionally an essential aspect of the anxiety circuit and is implicated in the pathophysiology of PTSD. Patients with PTSD exhibit a reduced hippocampal volume that is associated with severe symptoms. The hippocampus is an important structure in episodic reminiscence and spatial context encoding. Damage to the hippocampus leads to a reduction in reference encoding in people precisely as rodents. Neural circuits consisting of the hippocampus, amygdala and PFC are hypothetically required for contextual retrieval of anxiety memories after extinction. Disturbances in the functioning of the hippocampus, resulting in referential normalization in patients with PTSD, may determine patients to experience trauma-related symptoms again.

VNS in PTSD

Vagus nerve stimulation has shown promise as a therapeutic option in treatment-resistant obstructive disorders such as PTSD. Chronic VNS has been shown to limit anxiety in mice too and improve the Hamilton Anxiety Ranking Scale in patients struggling with treatment-resistant depression. After stimulation, the vagus nerve sends signals to the NTS and the NTS sends projections directly to the amygdala and hypothalamus. In addition, VNS enhances the projection of NE in the basolateral amygdala as well as the hippocampus and ventromedial prefrontal cortex. NE in the amygdala results in better extinction retention. Thus, VNS wants to be a true tool to increase extinction retention. For example, in mice, extinction retention paired with VNS therapy may cause fear and an increase PTSD like symptoms. In addition, VNS paired with extinction retention helps to facilitate plasticity between the ventromedial prefrontal cortex and the amygdala and leads to the extinction of conditioned fear responses.

Additionally, VNS can also increase extinction retention by helping to inhibit the effect of the sympathetic nervous system. It is possible that an immediate VNS-induced in anxiety disorders contributes to VNS driven extinction retention by assisting the CS to interfere with the sympathetic response, resulting in the CS's association with fear. However, randomized managed trials are needed to approve these comments.

One of the most sustained neurophysiological consequences of VNS is reduced hippocampus activity, through an increase of GABA secretion. As described above, the hippocampus is a quintessential component of the fear circuit, given that it is an important shape in episodic memory and spatial context encoding. A decrease in hippocampal activity after VNS has been cited in various studies of various conditions such as depression or schizophrenia.

The positive effect of nutritional components on PTSD

Emerging studies suggest that probiotics may be conceivable to reduce stress-induced inflammatory responses, as well as related symptoms. An investigative study of microbioma investigations of patients with PTSD and control of trauma exposure revealed that the survival of three microorganism lines in patients with PTSD was reduced: actinobacteria, with higher PTSD symptom scores. These microorganisms are essential for the immune system and their low abundance may contribute to immune system dysfunction and the development of PTSD symptoms. It is known about the use of a new model of immunization with heat-prepared

Mycobacterium vaccine which brought about a more active behavioral response than a psychological therapy. Studies conducted in nutritional volunteers have shown that the administration of one type of probiotics was associated with extended well-being, as well as a decrease in anxiety and psychological distress. These findings are all preliminary. A randomized double blind placebo control scientific studie aimed to explore the effect of controlled dietary supplements effect on microbioma signs and symptoms in patients with PTSD.

The positive effects of meditation and yoga on PTSD

Clinical evidence for the efficiency of *mindfulness-based stress reduction* (MBSR) in the treatment of PTSD. During MBSR, the gradual respiration and prolonged exhalation phase make the parasympathetic tone larger.

In addition, scientific studies have demonstrated the effectiveness of yoga as a therapeutic intervention for ablation of PTSD through a decline in stress response. Yoga practices in PTSD have led to additional reductions after anxious disorders. Yoga-responsive anxiety disorders, including PTSD, collectively go with low HRV and low GABA activity.

The interconnection of the PFC, hippocampus, and amygdala in combination with input from the autonomic nervous system and the GABA receptors presents a center through which symptoms can be reduced in addition to yoga-based practices. There are warning signs that conditioned anxiety reduction in PTSD is related to reduced PFC manipulation of amygdala activity. PFC activation, associated with extended parasympathetic activity at some point may increase inhibitory control over the amygdala via PFC, GABA activation; so it decreases amygdala over-activity in order to reduce PTSD symptoms.

The Science of IBD

Inflammatory bowel disorders are in most cases two disorders: ulcerative colitis (UC) and Crohn's disease (CD). IBD is a chronic, uncontrolled inflammation of the intestinal mucosa. The symptoms are: abdominal pain, diarrhea, fever, weight loss and severe urgency to have a bowel movement. In CD, the main symptoms are diarrhea, abdominal pain and weight loss, while in UC diarrhea is the predominant symptom most of the times accompanied by rectal bleeding.

Inflammatory bowel disorder affects approximately 1.5 million people in the United States and 2.2 million in Europe, and about 20% of IBD patients have a family history.In addition, industrialization led by the the free market will increase cases of IBD in Asia also.

There is increasing evidence that psychosocial work stressors in environmental exposure factors, including infections, western food diets and food additives, air and water pollution, capsules (antibiotics, hormones) and genetic elements (more than 250 genomics elements) are consistently identified in the pathogenesis of IBD, ultimately leading to a peculiar immune response to microbial exposure.

What distinguishes IBD from the inflammatory reactions seen in the everyday intestine is the inability to reduce inflammatory responses, such as when the gut turns to inflammation in response to a viable pathogen. Thus, inflammation is not reduced in humans with IBD, the mucosal immune system remains active for a long time, and the intestine remains inflamed for a long time. During inflammation, anti-inflammatory cytokines (IL-1 IL, IL-6, TNF) launched from the intestinal mucosa reach to VN afferent connections that terminate in the NTS, then intestinal data is sent to the HPA axis. Let's remember the great anti-inflammatory success of the vagus nerve which has been obtained via the cholinergic anti-inflammatory pathway(CAIP). As previously mentioned, ACh launched at the distal end of the VN efferent fibers reduces the production of pro-inflammatory cytokines such as TNF.

Over stimulation of VN may be an important step in the development of IBD.

VNS in IBD

It reflects the systemic inflammatory response to endotoxin and intestinal inflammation. The VN also regulates immune recreation of the spleen through connections with the splenic sympathetic nerve. In mice with colon inflammation, 3 h long daily VNS for a period of 5 days led to a decrease in inflammatory markers and an improvement in colitis symptoms.

Vagus nerve stimulation should be of activity in various inflammatory disorders, such as rheumatoid arthritis and some other TNF mediated diseases. In sufferers with rheumatism, a study that proved an increase of symptoms in the early and late stages of the disease showed that it occurred after 1or4 minutes daily appliance of VNS. This study was additionally done to show that VNS inhibits the formation of TNF and other cytokines in humans using the inflammatory reflex, thereby improving symptom severity. These facts argue for an anti-inflammatory role of the vagus nerve and present therapeutic remedies for patients with IBD.

Chapter 6: Causes of Anxiety, Depression And Inflammation.

Although it is the most well-known indication of mental distress in almost every nation on the planet, anxiety is often as a result of current Western social orders; Norman Mailer, for instance, proposed that "the regular job of twentieth-century man or woman is anxiety".

The idea of anxiety, in essence, was first brought to conspicuousness as a philosophical and psychoanalytic idea in the initial segment of the twentieth century. Freud was a major figure in the advancement of Western considering anxiety, which he thought about as a condition of inward pressure from which people are headed to getaway. At an essential level, anxiety is a sign to the sense of self (the part of the character that manages reality) that something overwhelmingly terrible is going to occur and that it needs to utilize a guard instrument accordingly.

Freud considered this to be getting from a newborn child's mental helplessness, which is a partner of its natural helplessness. People figure out how to adapt to anxiety incited by 'genuine' dangers, for example, the dread of being chewed by a canine, either by keeping away from circumstances prone to contain the risk or by physically pulling back from them. Freud's typology likewise included masochist anxiety emerging from an oblivious dread that we will lose control of libidinal motivations, prompting improper conduct, and good anxiety, emerging from dread of abusing our good or cultural codes. Moral anxiety, he recommended, shows itself as blame or disgrace.

The assignment of analysis is along these lines to fortify the capacity of the self-image to discover methods for adapting to anxiety, for example, 'disavowal', 'defense', 'relapse' (to a youth state) or 'projection'. Inside the existentialist philosophical custom, 'apprehension', from the German word for anxiety, is held to be a negative inclination emerging from the experience of human opportunity and obligation in this present reality where confidence and conventional social bonds have been undermined. Kierkegaard's exemplary case of existential apprehension is of an individual standing on the edge of a high bluff or working; alongside the dread of incidentally falling, the individual feels a nonsensical motivation to throw themselves over the edge on purpose.

The feeling the individual has after understanding that the person has this alternative is tension. Kierkegaard depicted the weight of settling on moral decisions as a result of freedom "the tipsiness of opportunity". Existential brain science along these lines continues from the assumption that anxiety originates from an emergency in the exercise of through and through freedom, which may be showed in anxiety about one's mortality, the certainty of loss, or about tolerating moral duty regarding one's considerations, emotions and activities.

That anxiety "some way or another feels new" might be clarified somewhat by the way that anxiety has been the subject of noteworthy logical research for not exactly 50 years, while the mental profession previously arranged diagnostic criteria for all the various disorders as of late as 1980, with the distribution of DSM-III. Resulting propels in diagnostic methods, combined with the improvement of successful pharmacological medicines and mental treatments, have provoked essential human services professionals to all the more promptly distinguish anxiety in their patients. Anxiety is currently perceived as one of the most pervasive mental medical issues in the UK.

Yet, there is great proof that it is still underreported, under-analyzed and under-treated. One explanation might be that, not normal for some other mental medical problems, individuals whose lives are influenced have not yet discovered a voice that verbalizes the full scope of encounters of anxiety, not only those of individuals living with anxiety disorders. As of late, this has started to change, as authors, bloggers and campaigners have furnished us with knowledge into "England's quiet plague" by depicting the anxiety, the complexities and subtleties of the different disorders and the impact that anxiety as upon their lives.

For instance, some people living with anxiety portray sentiments of disgrace and shame at their physical indications, such as profuse sweating which leads them to embrace what Freudian psychoanalysts would perceive as old-style guard systems: "they figure out how to close their anxiety from general visibility". As per Daniel Smith, "they figure out how to plug their anxiety inside themselves like a corrosive in a vial."

In any case, it works." Perhaps more altogether, the declaration of individuals living with anxiety bears us an increasingly adjusted energy about the job that it plays in molding their lives; as Scott Stossel, creator of My Age of Anxiety, puts it, "anxiety can be a spike to accomplishment just as a hindrance.

Picture a ringer bend with extraordinary anxiety on the extreme right and excessive absence of anxiety on the extreme left. If you're excessively on edge to where it's physically and mentally crippling, at that point your exhibition endures. In case you're not on edge enough, on the off chance that you're not locked in and marginally initiated by anxiety, so to speak, at that point your exhibition additionally endures." The voices of individuals living with the more intense types of anxiety help us to imagine anxiety as something more than essentially a condition that requires conclusion and treatment.

How people draw in with their anxiety, how they oversee it and speak to it to the more extensive world lifts anxiety past the domain of medicine and science and into a more extensive sociological and social setting.

What are the most well-known anxiety disorders?

Panic is a distortion of the body's ordinary reaction to dread, stress or fervor. Fits of anxiety are a time of extraordinary dread wherein manifestations grow unexpectedly and top quickly. Fits of anxiety have been depicted as a type of "enthusiastic short-circuiting" whereby the limbic brain all of a sudden assumes control over the body's working, prompting overpowering sensations, which may incorporate a beating heart, feeling faint, perspiring, flimsy appendages, sickness, chest torments, breathing uneasiness and sentiments of losing control.

Adrenaline overpowers the psychological capacities that would typically help the brain survey the actual reality of the danger to the body.

Fear is an extreme and unreasonable dread of a particular item or circumstance, with the end goal that it urges the individual to encounter it to try hard to maintain a strategic distance from it. Fears can be about unsafe things or circumstances that present a hazard; however, they can likewise be of innocuous circumstances, objects or now and then creatures. Social fear can incorporate a dread of being judged, investigated or embarrassed somehow or another.

It can show itself with a dread of doing certain things before others, for example, public speaking.

Although agoraphobia is often connected with a dread of open spaces, the principle include is extreme anxiety setting off a frenzy reaction in circumstances where help may not be promptly accessible; in fact, such emergencies often happen in restricted spaces. Individuals with agoraphobia seem to encounter two unmistakable kinds of anxiety— panic, and the anticipatory anxiety identified with dread of future fits of anxiety. Agoraphobia can have an emotional restricting impact upon the way of life of individuals living with the condition, as they try to maintain a strategic distance from circumstances that will put them on edge; for instance, just using areas they have known courses of escape like xits and fire escapes.

In outrageous cases, people are so dreadful they become homebound inside and out. Beginning of agoraphobia is for the most part between the ages of 18 and 35 and influences somewhere in the range of 1.5% and 3.5% of the overall public in its entirely created structure; in a less severe structure up to one of every eight individuals, for example around 7 million in the UK, might be upset by some agoraphobic side effects.

Post-Traumatic Stress Disorder (PTSD), or disorder, is a mental response to an exceptionally stressful occasion outside the scope of ordinary experience, for example, military battle, physical brutality, or a cataclysmic event. The manifestations, for the most part, incorporate depression, anxiety, flashbacks, intermittent nightmares, and shirking of circumstances that may trigger recollections of the occasion. One investigation of UK military workforce sent to Afghanistan found that of 1,431 members, 2.7% were named having likely PTSD. At the same time, a family unit overview of UK grown-ups assessed a commonness of 2.6% in men and 3.3% in ladies.

While the scope of studies researching the wellbeing difficulties of shelter searchers and displaced people have discovered that PTSD levels can be as much as multiple times higher than the age-coordinated overall public. A scope of stressors has been distinguished as affecting antagonistically on mental wellbeing, including that accomplished premigration, for example, torment, traumatic deprivation and detainment, yet in addition post-relocation factors, for example, separation, confinement, dejection and deferred basic leadership in the shelter procedure. One investigation of ladies' refuge searchers in Scotland, and Belgium found that 57% were over the cut-point for PTSD symptomatology.

Obsessive-Compulsive Disorder (OCD) influences around 2–3% of the population. It is described by undesirable, meddlesome, diligent or tedious musings, emotions, thoughts, sensations (fixations), or practices that make the sufferer feel headed to accomplish something (impulses) to dispose of the obsessive considerations. This gives transitory alleviation and not playing out the obsessive customs can cause incredible anxiety. An individual's degree of OCD can be anyplace from mellow to extreme, however on the off chance that severe and left untreated; it can crush an individual's ability to work at work, at school or even to lead an agreeable presence in the home.

Generalized Anxiety Disorder (GAD) is the most common analyzed anxiety disorder. Individuals with GAD think that it's difficult to control, to such a degree, that it infringes upon their day by day life. It makes sufferers feel on edge about a wide scope of circumstances and issues, instead of one explicit occasion. In contrast to a fear, which centers upon a particular person, place or circumstance, anxiety is pure diffusion of racing thoughts of impending disaster or events that have not occurred yet or did occur in the past, and overruns the sufferer's day by day life.

Although GAD is less severe than a fit of anxiety, its length and the mental and physical side effects, for example, crabbiness, poor fixation and the impacts of disturbed rest designs, imply that individuals with the disorder often think that it is hard to carry on with the existence they would want to live. Stray influences 2–5% of the populace and has expanded somewhat since 1993, yet represents as much as 30% of the mental medical issues in individuals seen by GPs, which clarifies why an analysis of individuals looking for help through essential consideration recommends a higher commonness pace of 7.2%.

Signs and symptoms of anxiety

Diagnosing uneasiness relies upon an individual's sentiments of stress so that manifestations will change. Character, co-happening emotional well-being conditions, and different variables may clarify an individual's side effects.

Anxiety can cause meddlesome or over the top contemplations. An individual with anxiety may feel bewildered or think that it's difficult to focus. Feeling fretful or baffled can likewise be an indication of uneasiness. Others with nervousness may feel discouraged.

Side effects of Anxiety can likewise be physical. Nervousness can cause excessively tense muscles or hyper Anxiety. Trembling, perspiring, a dashing heartbeat, discombobulation, and a sleeping disorder can also originate from Anxiety. Anxiety may even cause migraines, stomach related issues, trouble breathing, and sickness. On the off chance that physical manifestations of uneasiness are severe and unexpected, it might be a fit of anxiety.

What does anxiety resemble?

Individuals can give indications of uneasiness from numerous points of view. Some may turn out to be increasingly talkative, while others pull back or self-detach. Indeed, even individuals who appear to be cordial, agreeable, or brave can have Anxiety. Since Anxiety has numerous manifestations, what it looks like for one individual isn't the way it shows up for another.

Individuals who have nervousness might be pulled back; however, this isn't the situation for everybody with uneasiness. Now and then, uneasiness may trigger a "fight" instead of "flight" reaction, in which case an individual may seem angry. Bumbling over words, trembling, and nervous tics are regularly connected with nervousness. While they can show up in individuals with Anxiety, they are not always present, and a few people who don't have nervousness additionally give these indications.

On the off chance that you are uncertain on the off chance that somebody you know might be encountering nervousness, it may not be helpful to bring it up except if they do. Be that as it may, there are a few moves you can consider making on the off chance that you need to make an individual who may be on edge increasingly agreeable. You can:

- Be quiet with them

- Share inspirational statements or appreciation.

- Be unsurprising and be eager to impart subtleties to them if they inquire.

What does generalized anxiety mean?

Generalized Anxiety is otherwise called free-drifting Anxiety. It is recognized by ceaseless sentiments of fate and stress that have no immediate reason. Numerous individuals feel on edge about specific things, similar to cash, prospective employee meet-ups, or dating. However, individuals with free-coasting Anxiety can feel on edge for no unmistakable explanation. Generalized Anxiety can likewise mean excess of stress over a specific period of time.

The Diagnostic and Statistical Manual (DSM-5) distinguishes generalized anxiety disorder (GAD) as over the top stress that affects an individual on a practically everyday schedule. It should be most recent a half year or more and be hard to control. It should likewise not have the option to be better clarified by some other wellbeing condition. An individual determined to have GAD should also appear in any event three of the accompanying side effects:

- Frequent weakness

- Restlessness

- Irritability

- Difficulty centering

- Sleep issues

- Muscle strain

Numerous elements can add to free-coasting nervousness. Living in stressful or harsh situations might be a reason. In some cases, nervousness turns into a propensity. An individual used to feeling on edge about an occasion may continue feeling on edge once it is finished. A few therapists fight that advanced life causes free-coasting nervousness. As indicated by them, cutoff times, quick-paced ways of life, and staying aware of social media could create interminable Anxiety.

At the point when an individual can't discover where their anxiety originates from, therapy can help. Therapy regularly helps individuals get the hang of adapting abilities for managing side effects of stress. Aptitudes that help individuals with constant anxiety incorporate profound breathing, reflection, exercise, and individual correspondence.

WHAT CAUSES ANXIETY?

Anxiety, similar to the fight, flight, or freeze reaction, is for endurance. It enables individuals to secure themselves to evade hurt. Once in a while, an individual has elevated levels of anxiety routinely. They may feel helpless in managing their manifestations.

Both science and condition decide whether an individual will have anxiety. As it were, on edge conduct can be acquired, learned, or both. For instance, inquire about shows that on edge guardians are probably going to have on edge youngsters. Be that as it may, guardians may likewise display restless conduct. Assuming this is the case, they may impart that equivalent conduct in their kids. Having a stressful childhood can also expand an individual's odds of having anxiety. This is because anxiety turns into an approach to foresee risk and remain safe. Anxiety can likewise create because of uncertain trauma. Uncertain trauma may leave an individual in an elevated condition of physiological excitement. At the point when this is the situation, specific encounters can reactivate the old trauma. This is basic for individuals with posttraumatic stress (PTSD).

Types of anxiety

Anxiety is at the base of numerous emotional well-being conditions, including alarm assaults and fears. It is regularly legitimately identified with different conditions, similar to fixations and impulses, PTSD, and depression. Notwithstanding summed up anxiety, the DSM-5 records the accompanying emotional wellness issues as anxiety issue:

- Separation anxiety: Can be portrayed by hesitance to venture out from home or be separated from guardians and anxiety when isolated from parents and friends.

- Selective mutism: Selective mutism implies not talking at all in just a few circumstances. This may cause issues with scholastic, work, or social achievement.

- Panic: The Panic issue is analyzed by repeating alarm assaults, including physical indications of anxiety.

- Specific fears: Phobias are dread encompassing a particular person, circumstance, place or event which the individual keeps away from.

- Social anxiety: People with social anxiety feel dread or fear in social circumstances. The dread is frequently out of extent to the danger, and individuals with social anxiety may evade social circumstances.

- Agoraphobia: Agoraphobia is the fear of places and situations, enclosed spaces, going out and being in groups or using public transportation.

- Medication/substance-instigated anxiety: This condition is analyzed by stress that is by all accounts legitimately brought about by use of specific substances, similar to caffeine or liquor. The anxiety could likewise be brought about by a drug.

Chapter 7: How to Activate Your Vagus Nerve

It's clear that vagus nerve stimulation is important for optimal health. Although there is an FDA regulated device that you can have implanted in the body by sending electrical impulses to stimulate the vagus nerve, there are other natural ways of stimulating the vagus nerve without surgery, devices, or side effects.

These vagus nerve simple exercises that anyone can do but they work with consistency and action.

Positive Social Relationships - A study had participants think compassionately about others while silently repeating positive phrases about friends and family. Compared to the controls, the meditators showed an overall increase in positive emotions like serenity, joy, and hope after completing the class. These positive thoughts of others led to an improvement in vagal function as seen in heart-rate variability. The results also showed a more toned vagus nerve than when simply meditating.

Cold Exposure - Cold exposure such as cold showers or face dunking stimulates the nerve as well. Acute cold exposure has been shown to activate the vagus nerve and activate cholinergic neurons through vagus nerve pathways. Researchers have also found that exposing yourself to cold on a regular basis can lower your sympathetic "fight or flight" response and increase parasympathetic activity through the vagus nerve. Try finishing your next shower with at least 30 seconds of cold water and see how you feel. Then work your way up to longer periods of time. It's painful to do, but the lingering effects are worth it. You can also ease yourself into it by simply sticking your face in ice-cold water. Studies show that when your body adjusts to cold, your fight or flight (sympathetic) system declines and your rest and digest (parasympathetic) system increases–and this is mediated by the vagus nerve. Any kind of acute cold exposure including drinking ice cold water will increase vagus nerve activation.

Acupuncture - The ancient Chinese medicine treatment of acupuncture may be beneficial in stimulating the vagus nerve. Research shows that ear acupuncture can benefit the following: cardiovascular regulation, respiratory regulation, gastrointestinal tract regulation. Also, foot reflexology can decrease blood pressure by modulating the vagus nerve, according to a 2012 study.

Gargling - Another home remedy for an under-stimulated vagus nerve is to gargle with water. Gargling actually stimulates the muscles of the pallet which are fired by the vagus nerve directly. Pour yourself a cup of water. Take about a quarter cup (exact amount isn't important) and gargle it vigorously for 20-30 seconds. Swallow that water and take another quarter cup and gargle that 20-30 seconds. Keep repeating until all the water in the cup is gone. Repeat the above gargling exercise 3-4 times/day

Singing And Chanting - The vagus nerve is connected to your vocal cords and the muscles at the back of your throat. Humming, mantra chanting, hymn singing, and upbeat energetic singing all increase heart rate variability (HRV) in slightly different ways. Essentially, singing is like initiating a vagal pump sending out relaxing waves. Singing at the top of your lungs works the muscles in the back of the throat to activate the vagus. Singing in unison, which is often done in churches and synagogues, also increases HRV and vagus function. Singing has been found to increase oxytocin, also known as the love hormone because it makes people feel closer to one another. Compassion meditation has been shown to result in a more toned vagus nerve.

Massage - You can stimulate your vagus nerve by massaging your feet and your neck along the carotid sinus, located along the carotid arteries on either side of your neck. A neck massage can help reduce seizures. A foot massage help can lower your heart rate and blood pressure. A pressure massage can also activate the vagus nerve. These massages are used to help infants gain weight by stimulating gut function, largely mediated by activating the vagus nerve.

Laughter - Happiness and laughter are natural immune boosters. Laughter also stimulates the vagus nerve. Research shows how laughter increases HRV in a group environment. There are various case reports of people fainting from laughter and this may be from the vagus nerve/parasympathetic system being stimulated too much. Fainting can come after laughter as well as urination, coughing, swallowing or bowel movement - all of which are helped along by vagus activation.

Wave Vibration - Wave vibration has been heavily studied by the scientific community for its health benefits. This therapy involves standing on an oscillating plate that produces low-level vibrations. These vibrations then create positive stress throughout the body (like the kind of stress created by exercise). This stress activates the vagal nerve among other parts of the body.

Probiotics - Probiotics are an important part of the diet and are beneficial for many ailments from digestive problems to skin issues. It turns out, probiotics may also be helpful in stimulating the vagus nerve. Researchers of a 2011 study found that giving mice Lactobacillus Rhamnosus increased their GABA production and decreased stress as well as depression and anxiety-related behavior. Interestingly, those given the probiotics who did not have a vagus nerve did not see the same results. This suggests that the improved stress resilience had something to do with activation of the vagus nerve.

Healthy Fats and Omega-3s - Omega-3 fatty acids are essential fats that your body cannot produce itself. They are found primarily in fish and are necessary for the normal electrical functioning of your brain and nervous system. Salmon contains omega-3 fatty acids, which have been shown to stimulate the vagus nerve. They've been shown to help people overcome addiction, repair a "leaky brain", and even help reverse cognitive decline. Studies shown that they reduce heart rate and increase heart rate variability, which means they likely stimulate the vagus nerve. And high fish consumption is also associated with enhanced vagal activity and parasympathetic predominance.

Meditation and Neurofeedback - Meditation is my favorite relaxation technique and it can stimulate the vagus nerve and increase vagal tone. Research shows that meditation increases vagal tone and positive emotions, and promotes feelings of goodwill towards yourself. Another study found that meditation reduces sympathetic "fight or flight" activity and increases vagal modulation. OM chanting, which is often done during meditation, has also been shown to stimulate the vagus nerve. I couldn't find any research demonstrating this, but in my experience, neurofeedback significantly increased heart-rate variability and vagal tone as measured by EmWave2.

Yoga And Tai Chi - Both increase vagus nerve activity and your parasympathetic system in general. Studies have shown that yoga increases GABA, a calming neurotransmitter in your brain. Researchers believe it does this by stimulating vagal afferents (fibers), which increase activity in the parasympathetic nervous system. This is especially helpful for those who struggle with anxiety or depression. Studies show that tai chi also can enhance vagal modulation.

Breathing Deeply And Slowly - Your heart and neck contain neurons that have receptors called baroreceptors, which detect blood pressure and transmit the neuronal signal to your brain.

This activates your vagus nerve that connects to your heart to lower blood pressure and heart rate. Slow breathing, with a roughly equal amount of time breathing in and out, increases the sensitivity of baroreceptors and vagal activation. Deep and slow breathing is another way to stimulate your vagus nerve. It's been shown to reduce anxiety and increase the parasympathetic system by activating the vagus nerve. Most people take about 10 to 14 breaths each minute. Taking about 6 breaths over the course of a minute is a great way to relieve stress. You should breathe in deeply from your diaphragm. When you do this, your stomach should expand outward. Your exhale should be long and slow. This is key to stimulating the vagus nerve and reaching a state of relaxation. The best way to know if you're on the right track is by using the EmWave2 device. It's a biofeedback device that assists you in pacing your breathing.

Intermittent Fasting - Intermittent fasting can stimulate the vagus nerve. There are many health benefits to doing this. Intermittent fasting can boost your brain's growth hormone, improve mitochondrial function, and may help some people overcome brain fog and cognitive decline. Research also shows that fasting and caloric restriction increase heart rate variability, which is an indicator that it increases parasympathetic activity and vagal tone. The best way to start fasting is simply by eating dinner around 6, not eating anything after that before bed, and then eating a regular breakfast the next day. That should give you about 12-14 hours of fasting time.

Exercise - Exercise increases your brain's growth hormone, supports your brain's mitochondria, and helps reverse cognitive decline. But it's also been shown to stimulate the vagus nerve, which leads to beneficial brain and mental health effects. Walking, weightlifting and sprinting are the best forms of exercise, but you should choose a sport or exercise routine that you enjoy so that you'll stick with it consistently. Mild exercise also stimulates gut flow, which is mediated by the vagus nerve.

You don't have to be controlled by your body and mind. You have the power to tell them what to do. By stimulating the vagus nerve, you can send a message to your body that it's time to relax and de-stress, which leads to long-term improvements in mood, wellbeing, and resilience.

Increasing the vagal tone can significantly improve mood and reduce anxiety/depression as well as better manage them when they arise. Overall, It is hoped that the reader implements some of the basic steps in this book in your daily life, and you live more optimally.

Conclusion

One of the keys to dealing with anxiety is to learn how, through proper breathing, to stimulate your vagus nerve. The vagus nerve serves as the bridge between the mind and the body and regulates the reaction to relax. When performing diaphragmatic breathing with the partially closed glottis, you will relax the vagus nerve. Use your dead time to regularly use this technique and turn it into a routine, and the effects will amaze you.

The vagus nerve is the parasympathetic nervous system, an important element (the one that calms you down by controlling your response to relaxation).

It originates from the brainstem and is "wandering" all the way down into the abdomen, extending fibers to the tongue, pharynx, vocal chords, lungs, chest, liver, intestines, and glands releasing anti-stress enzymes and hormones (such as acetylcholine, prolactin, vasopressin, oxytocin), affecting appetite, metabolism and, of course, the calming reaction.

Vagus nerve acts as the connection between the mind and the body, and it is the cable behind the emotions and intestinal instincts of your heart. The key to managing your mental state and levels of anxiety can activate your parasympathetic system's calming nervous pathways.

This part of the nervous system cannot be managed on request, but you can partially activate the Vagus nerve by:

- Immerse your head in cold water (diving reflex)
- Trying to exhale against a blocked airway (Valsalva maneuver).
  - You can do this by holding your mouth shut and pinching your nose while trying to breathe out. It greatly increases the tension inside the chest cavity relaxing the Vagus nerve and increasing vagal tone
- Singing out loud
- And of course, **diaphragmatic breathing exercises**, strengthening the living nervous system will pay great dividends, and the best tool to do this is by exercising the body.

Appendix

https://en.wikipedia.org/wiki/Vagus_nerve

https://www.ncbi.nlm.nih.gov/pmc/articles/PMC5859128/

www.ingramcontent.com/pod-product-compliance
Lightning Source LLC
Chambersburg PA
CBHW031428210526
45464CB00005B/2106